VIBRANT LONGEVITY

Introducing You to *Total Approach Wellness and Aesthetics*

I0117202

VIBRANT LONGEVITY

Introducing You to *Total Approach Wellness and Aesthetics*

Cynthia Phillips, PAC
and Gerianne Geszler, MD

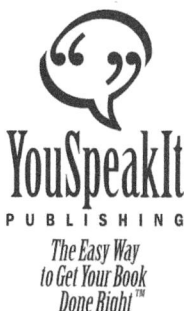

YouSpeakIt
PUBLISHING
The Easy Way
to Get Your Book
Done Right™

www.YouSpeakItPublishing.com

ISBN: 978-1-945446-57-3

Cynthia

There are many people I would like to thank. Gary Newton, pharmacist, who started this whole new way of thinking by inviting us to a seminar on bioidentical hormones. Eldred Taylor, MD, who got me out of the caterpillar line and started down a path to Wellness medicine instead of sickness medicine. Of course, my family and friends who put up with all my experimentation on them. I hope they are better for it.

Gerianne

To my mother, whose struggles for health led me to seek ways to help others not suffer with multiple health issues throughout their lives.

To my patients throughout the years, who helped open my eyes to their sufferings and encourage me to seek knowledge to guide them through their health journeys.

To my oldest son, Bart, who is the healthiest person I know, who nudged me along my journey to show me that food is the ultimate foundation for a healthy life.

Contents

Acknowledgments   9

Introduction   11

CHAPTER ONE

Taking Responsibility For Your Health   15

    Recognize You Have A Problem   15

    Playing Russian Roulette With Your Health   21

    The Willingness To Change   26

CHAPTER TWO

Confusion About What To Follow   33

    So Many Experts, How Do You Decide?   33

    Treatment Must Be Research Based   38

    All Food And Vitamins Are Not Equal   42

CHAPTER THREE

Live Well And Feel Well   49

    Aging: You Don't Have To Feel Bad   49

    How Do You Accomplish Aging Well?   56

    Doing The Things You Want To Do   61

CHAPTER FOUR

Emotional Health Is A Critical Element   65

    Negative Emotions Can Boycott

       Your Overall Health   65

    How To Manage Stress   69

    Dealing With Unresolved Trauma   73

CHAPTER FIVE

Why Exercise Is Important   81

Everyone Can Exercise   81

How To Pick The Correct Exercise   87

More Is Not Necessarily Better   93

Conclusion   101

Next Steps   103

About The Authors   105

Acknowledgments

We would like to thank many people who have contributed to this book. It is an accumulation of more than sixty years of experience that has brought us to this point today. Starting from most recent, the support team at YouSpeakIt Publishing and Freedom Practice Coaching that brought them to us. We never would have considered writing a book had they not made it such an organized process.

Thanks to Debbie Lallier, of Haymount Healing and Wellness, for suggesting we do this. Over the years, we have accumulated an inordinate amount of knowledge, but we never knew how to gather it together to make sense to our readers. Debbie helped us to recognize ourselves as resources with something to share.

A special thank you to all our professors and mentors over the years and the researchers who have pioneered this new movement into metabolic medicine. We have stepped away from the *normal* way of thinking and become pioneers of the future of medicine. Thank you for giving us the courage to embark on this wonderful journey called *Wellness*.

To all the functional medicine providers who have braved the mainstream medical paradigm and suffered not only ridicule but ostracism to help change the paradigm of health—thank you for helping us feel strong in the knowledge that there is a better way, and that healing is usually obtainable with natural therapies instead of pharmaceuticals.

To all our patients in the past and in the future who have taken or will take this journey with us: you are the ones who have inspired us to continue this journey and create this book.

Introduction

After having a severe allergic reaction to Amoxicillin while in school, Cynthia's health went downhill, and she was unable to find someone to help her. She then began the journey to *fix herself*. She knew traditional medicine had caused the problem but could not fix it, so she started on a ten-year journey to learn all she could about the complicated body systems and correct what was going wrong.

Because of this experience, Cynthia has a passion to help as many people as she can because she relates to the hopelessness they are feeling. She has dedicated herself to their problems and finding the answers to make them feel better. This is why she does what she does. This is why she chose to practice metabolic medicine. Cynthia elected to get back to the basics and find out *why* health is declining and try to reverse this, not just cover up the symptoms.

Dr. Gerianne Gezler is committed to the functional medicine approach because she has seen how traditional medicine has failed so many of her friends and associates over the years. She has witnessed patients, family, and associates stricken with serious illnesses that very well may have been prevented and possibly reversed with a comprehensive holistic approach. Seeing how the insurance model has let down so many people drives her passion to help people to shift their paradigm from relying on pharmaceuticals into a partnership with her patients to travel a healing journey.

She always tries to practice what she preaches and strives to incorporate an active lifestyle with clean eating and a healthy spiritual awareness.

This book is for you. It takes you on a journey to examine all facets of health. It would be a struggle to achieve health without considering all of them. We wrote this book as a guideline—a starting point—to inspire you to gain a foothold on vibrant longevity. We hope you will become empowered and begin your journey toward optimal wellness after reading this book.

Our book is about our wellness journey experiences, both personally and professionally. We have included information about five elements that are most important for you to understand on your journey to wellness. Because this journey can be overwhelming when you start, we have included a helpful overview of the journey and suggestions for how you can accomplish it.

We wrote this book to share our medical philosophies with our patients—past, present, and future. It is difficult in a few hour-long appointments to let you know who we are and what we are about. We hope through this book you will see how we feel about what we teach and how much we want to educate you about a healthier lifestyle. Our expertise and knowledge come from self-experience, sacrifices, and dedication.

Because everyone is different, a rigid guide to wellness is not helpful. Therefore, this book is written for you to use as a general guide to modify for your specific needs as you see fit. You do not have to start at the beginning and read every word we have written. As you journey toward wellness, read the section that speaks to you at the time. If your main struggle is with exercise, read the section on exercise first. If you feel you need to know more about vitamins or are confused about which vitamins to take, start with Chapter Two. We do not give you specifics but instead, give you suggestions to guide you in making choices that fit your problem or lifestyle.

We do not expect you to use this book as an all-inclusive reference, but to use it as a guide on your journey to optimal wellness.

We have put a lot of thought, dedication, and education into this guide and our wellness program. We want you to be motivated, dedicated, and, in the end, feel so good that you will want to share your experience with the ones you love, your friends, and even casual acquaintances. We hope your mental and physical experiences are so positive you will want to tell everyone about your incredible wellness.

Remember, the entire reason for this lifestyle program is to get you back to the best version of yourself. When you feel good, you can play with your children, your grandchildren, and your great grandchildren. You can take that cruise you've been saving for in retirement, whereas before, you may not have had the vibrant health to go.

If your goal is to be able to play in the park with your children or grandchildren, lift them over your head, run with them, or simply take them shopping, then you need to be healthy. We want you to have the energy, happiness, and well-being to live your life. As parents ourselves, we know how important it is to feel good, so you can participate in family life. We want you to enjoy your life and achieve your goals.

CHAPTER ONE

Taking Responsibility for Your Health

In the long run, we shape our lives,
and we shape ourselves.
The process never ends until we die.
And the choices we make are ultimately
our own responsibility.
~ Eleanor Roosevelt

RECOGNIZE YOU HAVE A PROBLEM

We have both worked in busy primary care offices for over twenty-five years and have heard the same things said over and over again. Many people come into the office with complaints of fatigue, their legs are swelling, they don't sleep—just a litany of problems. Patients usually want a pill to fix everything. Then, when they get the pill, they have side effects and they feel worse.

We find this traditional approach to be both very frustrating for us professionally and for the patients personally. We elect to discuss with patients how they can alter their lifestyle to help their problems.

Unfortunately, most of the time the response is something like: *Oh, I could never do that.*

As providers with a foundation in functional medicine, when we hear the ways in which people are stuck, it's frustrating because we know that we could help them. We know the patients who listen to our coaching and apply the information we share feel much better. Unfortunately, in our fast-paced world, many people go with the litany of excuses, instead of taking responsibility for their health.

Are Little Issues Creeping Up on You?

Many people become so wrapped up in their everyday activities, they ignore the signals their body is sending them. When their systems fail to function optimally, causing feelings of fatigue, they discount those feelings as simply getting older.

Or, perhaps people begin to gain weight and think: *That's what happens with age.*

For others, the start of aches and pains—*Well,* they figure, *that's only part of the process.*

Many people accept these health issues as natural and expected symptoms of aging.

That's the real issue, right—health problems creeping up on you?

Many years ago, one of our patients filled out our functional medicine questionnaire and she said, "My gosh, I didn't realize I had so many symptoms."

Another patient, after starting bioidentical hormones, thyroid medication, and vitamins, said, "I didn't realize how bad I felt until I started feeling better."

So, many people initially ignore much of what is going on within their body. They're not in tune with their bodies until they are suddenly diagnosed with diabetes, cancer, or some other disease. But, what they do not realize is that disease is a slow progression; it doesn't happen overnight. There are usually subtle changes in lab results or physical changes that are predictors of more serious potential disease when recognized early in the disease process.

Is Your Busy Life Consuming You?

Remember to watch out for excuses, such as:

- *I've worked long hours and don't have time to shop for good quality food.*
- *My kids play sports so we're never home.*
- *I don't have time to prepare a meal; we can grab fast food.*

Excuses keep you from taking responsibility for your health. All of us can rearrange our time. For example, you can get up an hour earlier in the morning or prepare dinners during the weekend. There are little changes you can make in your routines that translate into a large difference in your health.

We must prioritize our health. Especially as parents, we can get caught up in our kids' activities and set aside our health, so kids can play a sport or join a club. Or, people work two jobs so they can have a new kitchen instead of taking care of the one body they have. Prioritizing your health is better than compromising it for a remodeled room, a new car, or whatever other materialistic good that you might want.

It is important to eat healthy foods, feel the sunshine, smell the roses, and experience nature. The fast-paced productivity and material-driven world we live in can be a great distraction. So many people forget to catch their breath and reflect on what is important, until it's too late.

Are You in Denial About Your Health?

A close friend and colleague always said he felt good, but he never exercised. He never challenged himself more than walking from his car to his office.

Had he challenged himself with routine exercise, he would have recognized the subtle signs of declining health. Unfortunately, he died much too soon.

Some people come to accept dysfunction in their body instead of being proactive and delving into why it is happening. They don't seek a functional medicine provider who will find the cause; instead, they continue to tolerate the dysfunction. Many people don't use their bodies much.

We've heard patients say things like: *Well, I felt fine, and then suddenly I had breast cancer.*

Or they *suddenly* have a heart attack or stroke.

Even if you never walk around the block and all you do is sit on the couch and eat chips or other junk food, you might feel fine. But, if you're not doing anything with your body except walking to the kitchen, you're not asking your body to function as intended.

We recommended trying a fitness tracker to a patient who was surprised when she initially netted her steps.

How many steps was she taking?

Maybe 2000? Maybe 900?

Her average was 600 in a day. She was flabbergasted that she moved so little and continued to wear her tracker. About three months later, she came to our office. She had gotten all the way up to 5,000 steps a day and thought that was an amazing accomplishment. We did too.

Sometimes, people are in denial about their health, not because they want to be, but because they don't know how bad it is. They have no comparison. Some people are isolated in their houses—just like our client who tried the fitness tracker. She was isolated, so initially she didn't know that the mere 600 steps a day of movement wasn't very much. Once she recognized how her lack of movement was affecting her health, she had to face it. She couldn't deny it anymore, and she did something about it.

People often assume they are healthy solely because they have not been diagnosed with a disease. We've heard people who have hypertension and are on a statin say they're healthy because their vital signs or lab results are in the normal range.

When your numbers are good, you're glad. But, are you in a state of optimal wellness?

Reflect on when you have felt your best:

- When did you feel vibrant and alive?
- Think back to that time and ask yourself: *How do I feel now, compared to then?*
- At your age, do you feel that you are at your optimal health?
- Do you feel that declining health is a normal part of aging?

In other words, don't resign yourself to a life of discomfort or disability as a natural part of aging.

Some of our patients in their seventies say things like: *I'm seventy-four; what do you expect? I'm not going to get up and move off the couch; I'm old.*

But again, this is because they are in denial about their health. There are ninety-year-olds who run marathons. It's all a matter of perception when it comes to your health. It is important to self-reflect and look upon those your age who have achieved optimal health as mentors. Listen to what they say, and always strive to be the healthiest for your age. You want to strive to be your best. Don't settle for the status quo.

PLAYING RUSSIAN ROULETTE WITH YOUR HEALTH

One of our patients was a seventeen-year-old girl with high cholesterol and prediabetes. She did not eat well and she admitted it. We told her that at this point in her life, at only seventeen, she could prevent disease. She could keep herself from becoming like her mother—who had diabetes, hypertension, and high cholesterol—if she would just take the opportunity at this point to change her lifestyle.

Our patient said, "I eat crap, I want to continue eating crap, and I don't want to change my diet. Give me a pill to make me better."

We don't want any of our readers or patients to adopt the attitude of this person. We want them to recognize at this point in their lives—the earlier the better—it's better to prevent a disease than to try to reverse a disease. We especially want our patients to avoid preventable diseases.

Hippocrates said twenty-four hundred years ago, "Everyone has a physician inside him or her, we just have to help it in its work. The natural healing force within each one of us is the greatest force in getting well."

It's Easier to Prevent Than to Reverse

If you start with a healthy lifestyle at a young age, you have a better chance of preventing disease and living a healthy life. You can continue a healthy lifestyle and address health issues with simple interventions, such as supplements, exercise, or detoxification. You should be able to avoid long-term dependence on pharmaceutical medications or surgeries.

We have advanced testing capabilities to look for vitamin and hormonal deficiencies and intestinal tract abnormalities. Basic tests can detect conditions we can easily reverse with some lifestyle changes or supplements. Simple changes can make a difference in preventing disease before it becomes a disease process.

Genetic alterations can cause certain vitamin deficiencies, a phenomenon we can determine by testing patients at an early age. It is even possible to lessen or prevent the effects of depression that can be caused by vitamin deficiencies, diabetes, or poor gut health. It's vital that you become knowledgeable about what's going on in your body, so that you can hopefully reverse those things before they become a large problem and translate into disease.

Some conditions can be reversed if they are detected at an early stage. You can have some really good results, for example, with Type 2 diabetes. A person does not develop diabetes overnight. It takes years of exhausting their insulin supplies before their pancreas fails to produce enough insulin to process their sugar. There is time to take proactive steps to make lifestyle changes.

However, when more serious events occur, like a stroke or heart attack, you can't reverse those events. A part of your body has died. Surgery to install coronary stents or bypasses are very painful and expensive interventions to *prevent* catastrophic events such as strokes or heart attacks, but they do not address the root causes. Unfortunately, many people hear about lifestyle changes only after they have had these procedures. It is far better to avoid the need for surgery altogether by embarking on a plan to improve your health, the earlier the better. Your body has an amazing ability to protect and repair itself, but if you've exhausted your reserves, you don't have the ability to rebuild, resupply, and strengthen.

You Can't Do All the Research Yourself

There's so much health information on the internet, and it's very easy to get caught up in someone's advertising hype, especially if it makes promises about results that sound good. Unless you received the training to understand the medical research, you could end up traveling down the wrong path, wasting many years and dollars, and maybe doing yourself harm. Many people think they are eating a healthy diet based on magazine articles, self-help books, or TV programs, but they keep gaining weight, gaining weight, gaining weight. They come for a consultation, and we look at their weight struggle and find out they are eating a completely skewed and poorly balanced diet.

There is a lot of misinformation available to the public. It takes a person qualified in the principles of functional medicine to glean the information that's there. Find someone who can define what is hype or a fad and what will help you get down to the basics. There's no one diet or exercise program that will fit all.

So, when you do research yourself, you might come upon a plan or program that makes you think: *Oh my gosh, that's the best thing for me,* but in reality, the *best thing* will probably be some variation of it.

As your qualified coaches, we consider you as an individual and look at the whole you. We don't view you through the lens of possible monetary gain; we do not compare you to what a similar population of people looking at the internet might spend their money on. Our goal is to provide you with the education and knowledge with which you can make appropriate lifestyle changes.

Lifestyle medicine is an individualized process. Be skeptical of what you hear or read. It's easy to become confused. Besides media marketing for products, there are chat groups and blogs that can lead you down paths of misinformation.

Becoming Informed by a Qualified Coach or Mentor

When a qualified health professional looks at your life and your lifestyle from many aspects, they can analyze what is going on with your health and guide you in the right direction. And, like doing the research yourself when choosing a diet, when you do pick a coach or mentor, you need to make sure that person is qualified. A lot of practitioners open so-called "functional medicine clinics" because functional medicine, as well as the use of bioidentical hormones, have become fashionable buzzwords.

There are many people who are not qualified to be your coach. There are several institutes dedicated to the education of healthcare practitioners that focus on functional, metabolic, and regenerative medical sciences. To assure you have a qualified healthcare practitioner look for designations such as American Board of Anti-Aging/Regenerative Medicine

(ABAARM) or Institute for Functional Medicine (IFM) certifications. Also, look for reviews about them.

If there are a lot of people writing reviews like: *They took me in, they were good, and they did a great job*, then they would probably be a good coach. A referral from a person who has been to that coach or mentor is a good way to be certain that they will also be of help to you.

A coach or clinician needs to engage with you, and you as a patient need to be empowered. Your coach and you must work together to stay on the same page. You need to get together, get along, and have the same goals. Additionally, you need to choose somebody you feel comfortable with in setting mutual goals for your health, someone you're comfortable with while discussing your health issues and asking questions.

THE WILLINGNESS TO CHANGE

Recall the example of the seventeen-year-old patient who was prediabetic. It would not matter if she had come into a functional medicine practice or to see a coach because she was not open or willing to change.

When you go down the path of a lifestyle change it is essential that you:

- Keep your mind open to new ideas
- Be willing to try new things
- Devote yourself to making the change

Otherwise, no treatment plan will be successful.

We really want to help people and we really want them to help themselves. We want our patients to be empowered and improve their health. This is our passion. We're not doing this for the money, that's for sure. We are doing it because we really believe a healthy lifestyle is critical for optimal wellness and disease prevention, and we practice what we preach. We demand the same healthy lifestyle for ourselves.

Reflect on Your Health

The importance of self-reflection is something that we can't overemphasize. Most Americans do not reflect much on their health until something goes wrong. The following encounter with a patient illustrates this point.

A woman needed a hip replacement.

The patient said, "You know, I'm in pretty good health, and I don't think I want to have surgery, so I'm going to hold off."

We concurred, saying, "Well, you never want to have surgery unless you absolutely have to."

The patient stood up and started walking, revealing a severe limp. She said, "It's because I am cleaning my house up for spring. Normally, I don't do that much activity."

This is a prime example that shows if you're not active, you're not going to have optimal health. Housecleaning for this patient was so stressful that her hip was bothering her.

If you're not using your body to its fullest potential, what good is it?

You only have one body and you need to take care of it. You can't get another one, you can't replace it. If you're not really paying attention to the signals your body gives you, then you are missing out on those subtle signs that something is not working. Many subtle signs, such as inflammation, appear when you don't take care of your health. These signs let you know of evolving issues that need to be addressed.

Be Honest With Yourself

Denial is a powerful defense tool. There are so many excuses people can create about their health. Reflecting on your health is essential, but in order for this to be helpful, you must be honest with yourself. If you can't be honest, reflecting on your own health will only be an illusion.

We invite you to open your eyes and take a loving—but real—look at yourself. Many people need a life event, such as an injury they can't recover from quickly, to inspire them to make changes.

Events like this can be enough to self-examine and ask: *Am I truly healthy? Why did I not recover from this event as fast I should?*

Or, maybe you get a cold or pneumonia, and you notice your co-worker recovered within five days but it took you fifteen days, or you ended up in the hospital. At that point, you need to reflect on your health and wonder why your immune system is not helping you get over that illness.

It is much easier to deny declining health than it is to admit it because sometimes admitting it means you need to face these challenges. Once you realize you are having challenges with your health, you must figure out what to do, or seek help for what to do. It can feel easier in the short term to bury your head in the sand and ignore the signals—hold your hands over your ears and eyes and not pay any attention to what's going on with your body.

Knowledge is power, but you must use that knowledge. Many people don't even want the knowledge. They just want to continue to deny their health problems because they think it's easier to stay on the same path. It feels much harder to change.

Open Yourself Up to a New Way of Thinking

When we hold seminars, one of the main issues we address is traditional medicine and what it can, and cannot, do for you. Traditional medicine is what we are all used to in America. We know that when you get a disease, there is a medicine. Television advertising tells us this. Lots of commercials tell us exactly what medicine we need for each disease.

Consider the direct marketing of prescription-only medications to the viewing masses. One in particular, Repatha—which touts a 71 percent reduction in *bad* cholesterol—seems quite impressive, but advertisers fail to stress these results are in conjunction with the use of a high-dose statin. And, oh yes—the cost is approximately $12,000 to $15,000 per year.

But, functional medicine is not that way. As a patient, if you open yourself up to different possibilities unfamiliar to you and treatments not mainstream, you will be introduced to a whole new realm of healing possibilities.

People often validate their perceptions with comments they hear on TV. There are currently several televised programs that at least address functional medicine cures. A while ago, one such show had a segment on vitamin D. Previously, vitamin D was not widely accepted

Similarly, years ago, fish oil used to be considered quackery.

People wondered: *What the heck is fish oil going to do for anybody?*

But, once it got on TV, people started seeing in it in magazines, and, as it was promoted, people began opening up to it. You must allow yourself to be ahead of the curve and be open to some of these treatments. It often seems that the treatments in functional medicine are new, but they're really not. They've been used for a long time and they're coming back into common awareness as they are backed by scientific research.

With a functional medicine approach, we revive our basic chemistry. It addresses the things that are going on in our bodies every day. Much of functional medicine, such as knowing about vitamin D and fish oil, has been ten to twenty years ahead of mainstream medicine. Trust the process and remember, you must trust the person who is guiding you. Your health mentor must be someone who is researching, going to seminars, and listening to other people who are at the forefront of the functional medicine empowerment.

I started the Total Wellness program with Dr. Geszler mid-June of 2017. Just six months later, I have experienced significant changes.

Here are just a few of these changes:

- *Lost close to thirty pounds—a 30 percent decrease in body fat*
- *Reduced blood pressure from the yellow zone to green (reduced blood pressure 10–20 points)*
- *Reduced coffee from four to five cups a day to one*
- *Totally rid of heartburn*
- *Increased energy and stamina*
- *Decreased use of asthma inhaler*
- *Decreased sugar and junk food cravings*
- *Workout routine resulting in increased strength and muscle mass*

~ David M.

CHAPTER TWO

———————

Confusion About What to Follow

Those who think they have no time for healthy eating . . .
will sooner or later have to find time for illness.
~Edward Stanley

SO MANY EXPERTS, HOW DO YOU DECIDE?

Lots of companies have vitamins, supplements, or diets promising you energy, focus, memory, weight loss, virility, hair growth, and to cure bowel problems. However, it's confusing to know what's right for you, so most people search the internet. When they do, they become more confused.

How do you integrate all the information and decide which method you want to use?

We can provide guidelines for how to research and interpret the information and what steps to take to dispel any myths or fallacies. You want to look at a method that will empower you to take charge of your health. What you really want is the long-term fix.

Don't Trust an Advertisement

The concept of *well-being*—which refers not only to the absence of disease, but also includes lifestyle behavior choices to ensure health, avoid preventable diseases and conditions, and to live in a balanced state of body, mind, and spirit—is all over the internet and television. Many of the self-proclaimed *well-help* experts have no scientific knowledge or background and are all too often profit driven. So, when you are deciding whether to believe a claim, be careful. Remember, you want to choose information that empowers your health, and you need to avoid getting caught up by the advertising hype.

Everyone selling health products claims to be an expert. We want to help you bust through the myths and false information that you are exposed to. Every day, we are bombarded with advertisements on TV, the internet, and magazines. Advertisements tout that their products are the newest and greatest, best things.

It's easy to become caught up in the hype of a slick advertisement that tells you things like: *We have the best weight loss pill,* or *this is the best vitamin to make you strong and give you virility.*

It isn't easy to know if the quality of a health product has been researched, or if it's made by someone who's more interested in making money than in providing health. Some of our patients come in with long lists of sundry supplements that they've picked up through the years, but their regimens never seem to come together in any sort of systematic form.

When we ask our patients how they decided which supplements and vitamins to take, the answer is often "from advertisements." They read an article and they decided to try this or that, or they heard an ad and it sounded like something for them. Before long, they end up with a two-page list of daily supplements, but they don't feel any better.

Celebrity Endorsement Doesn't Make It Viable

Celebrities offer testimonials about the effectiveness of many different health products. The biggest-selling product they testify about is weight-loss systems.

So, the question for you to ask is: Why give credibility to a celebrity who is promoting a short-term fix?

In our many years of observing various celebrity-promoted weight-loss systems, we find most of the people who used them have gained their weight back. Celebrities often try to endorse good products, but much of the time they don't have experts and quality research behind them.

You must look at the celebrities who have collaborated with experts, such as dietitians and nutritionists. The doctors who have been studying weight-loss medicine for a long time will have a much better product to bring to the public, and the celebrity is there just to give it attention.

There are advocates for just about every style of eating possible: all fruit, all vegetables, all meat; and this, that, and the other. Sometimes, a person will become attracted to one of those systems because it works for them, and they think it's going to be easy to stay on it. For instance, if your chosen program ships preplanned meals to you and you don't have to think about it, then hey—that's wonderful! This type of prepackaged diet attracts many kinds of people.

Yet, when you consider excess weight as a symptom of many things going wrong in the body, an easy fix probably won't work long term. Every problem in the body is related to multiple dysfunctions. Don't rely on one celebrity who has little knowledge of how to fight disease and regain health.

Do Your Research and Get Testimonials

Many experts are nothing more than self-proclaimed experts. They give advice on diet and vitamins with little scientific research backing their claims. If you seek care from someone, it is prudent to investigate that person to ensure they have some sort of formal education *beyond* their medical training.

If possible, speak to others who have been helped. We did this independently and were amazed at what we found. There are many so-called experts who might have studied and tried out some things in their particular field. And then, they claim that they have done the research and done their homework, but that is not the same as having expertise.

When checking to learn if someone has expertise, read the reviews from people who have tried their system or worked with them, then look for multiple good reviews. This is one way to see if the practitioner has succeeded. Then, you can have some assurance that the system is a good system. For example, if you buy electronics online, you probably read the reviews. You look at what the customer testimonials say to see if the equipment you want to buy worked well, if it was a good value, and if the customers are happy with the result.

If you see multiple reviews that say things like: *Yes, this was great, it was wonderful,* and then one person who says something like: *No, it was a piece of junk,* then you know most people gave it a good review.

You must do the same thing when regarding health systems. If many people tried it and achieved good results from it, then it probably is a good product or system.

Many people misperceive the knowledge that physicians and providers have when they have completed training. People expect providers to know how to track down a lot of common symptoms that may be related to multiple-organ hormonal dysfunctions. You may be surprised to find out that this information is not given to us as students during our medical school education. Medical school is pharmaceutically driven, and most research is pharmaceutically derived. You must find a practitioner who is willing to acquire that knowledge on their own.

TREATMENT MUST BE RESEARCH BASED

Traditional medicine is probably ten to twenty years behind the research. Functional medicine is ahead of the curve of maintaining health and treating many different health issues. You must be careful that the practitioner guiding you is basing their decisions on research. For example, we could say we were thyroid experts and take an approach to treatment that is not research based—there are so many products and programs being marketed for thyroid health from which to choose.

Some diet recommendations in the past were not based on research. The low-fat, low-cholesterol diet was not research based. Cholesterol being the primary cause of heart disease and statin drugs making you live longer after a heart attack— much of this is very controversial because of the quality of the research.

Additionally, the determination that testosterone replacement therapy causes prostate cancer was not research based. It was based on three patients in an esoteric 1941 article buried deep within the archives of Harvard's medical library. A study presented at the American Urological Association annual meeting in 2016 showed that testosterone treatment does not increase prostate cancer risk.

These are two examples that the entire country has embraced and endorsed yet were not based on research. Unfortunately, this position went on to be taught in medical schools without challenge.

One Answer Does Not Make a Complete Picture

Your best defense against hype and inadequate research is to be an informed consumer. You must remember this as you try to wade through all the information and misinformation. Because everyone is different, everyone has a different problem, and the solutions will probably be different. It is vital for you and your provider to view your health issue as a complete picture and not narrow your quest for total health to one specific symptom.

Perhaps you have weight gain, and you treat only the weight. Or, you have headaches and you take something for the pain. If you try a fad diet or a fad treatment, all you are doing is treating one symptom and not looking at the body as a whole. You may be missing an underlying problem. All the parts and systems of the body need to be working together for optimal wellness.

If you have a symptom such as fatigue, the cause is most likely not just your adrenals, or your thyroid, or your B_{12} level—it could also be the microbes in your gut, for instance. There is rarely one answer to a big problem. As you begin to repair the abnormalities that you find in different body systems, a healthy person will emerge with lessening symptoms.

You may even forget what your symptoms initially were, and think back: *Oh yeah, I didn't used to feel well!*

You Can't Do the Research if You Don't Have the Background

It's very challenging to research health problems without a medical background. Even if answers are to be found, many times they are only partial. If the person doing the research is a layperson, they won't have the ability to do any kind of testing to further look at the problem. When people research their own issues, we they often get tunnel vision and only focus on the one problem that they've latched onto.

Even we use the internet at times, looking for something minor. Some information is hard to find and we end up searching all over the place. Chronic Lyme disease has largely been discounted by traditional medicine but emerging research is finding it to be a significant condition. Fibromyalgia causes have also been highly researched. It seems to be a *garbage-can diagnosis*, in which practitioners cannot identify the cause of debilitating pain. When a health problem becomes popularized, there is often an explosion of websites offering advice.

So, how do you go about organizing all the information on the internet to use effectively as a treatment?

You Need Someone Who Can Sort Out Research Hype

It is difficult to be totally objective about your own healthcare issues. If you are given a tool to make a framework for healthy living, you can then empower yourself to improve and achieve long-term, optimal health. It is a rare individual who can sort things out themselves and come up with a solution. Even in our own clinic, we try not to treat ourselves. Although we have medical knowledge and a lot of information, we don't see things in ourselves that others see.

It takes someone else to see you from the outside, who can look at you completely, to be able to understand what's going on. Sometimes, you don't want to think that you have a problem, so you might minimize the symptoms, but when someone else looks at you, they don't do that. They can see through that because they don't have the bias.

When you go to another practitioner and fill out their extensive symptom questionnaire, you may see many things that you hadn't realized had implications for your health. Again, looking at one little piece of research, you might go down the wrong path for what you've decided is your diagnosis. That's why you need someone objective to help you get there.

ALL FOOD AND VITAMINS ARE NOT EQUAL

Vitamins are not regulated. Our food sources are definitely not regulated, and a lot of people will try fad diets. Many people will take vitamins when they don't know the source. Indeed, we have found that most patients don't consider the source when picking and choosing what vitamins or supplements to take. But, it's vital to know the ingredients and their origin because it can make all the difference in the patient's outcome. Quality, purity, and bio-availability are very important and should be consistent. Consumer Labs tests over-the-counter supplements and frequently finds that they do not contain the amount on the label, if any at all. They may also contain additional fillers that may be hazardous.

Consider Your Source

Many people assume that all over-the-counter (OTC) supplements contain what the labels say they do. Since they are not regulated, independent organizations are often called upon to determine their compliance. Consumer Labs is one such organization that periodically tests different OTC supplements and publish their reports. The group often finds a small percentage of the labeled ingredients in the pill or capsule, but additionally, many OTC supplements are contaminated with toxins and even irradiated.

Many ingredients from China are highly contaminated with toxins. If you can't trust the company supplying you with supplements and vitamins, you may be doing more harm than good. The company that you buy supplements from needs to be trustworthy. Many companies are not trustworthy because the temptation to make a lot of money causes them to compromise quality in the process of manufacturing and selling vitamins. Ideally, you want the supplements you purchase to be verified compliant by the National Sanitation Foundation (NSF) and Therapeutic Goods Administration (TGA).

Because OTC supplements don't have to be regulated, vitamin sources are rarely investigated. Many vitamins are made using synthetic ingredients. In contrast, the whole-food ingredient is usually a much better source. You also get better value and nutrition from supplements sourced responsibly from whole food. This is the way your body absorbs it—the way your body recognizes it. It's the same thing with your food.

If you have lots of foods in your diet derived from genetically modified organisms (GMOs), your body may not recognize what you're eating and not use the nutrients the way it should. As much as possible, you should look for foods that are non-GMO.

It takes research to learn which foods are GMOs, and you must become informed. We've done a lot of that research ourselves. We have discovered that some of the sources that we initially thought were good—for instance, our turmeric—was contaminated with lead. So, it's hard to know. It's even hard for us, as much as we know. We must constantly consider sources, and the quality of ingredients they use.

Pharmaceutical-Grade Nutraceuticals

Pharmaceutical-grade standards, according to the Food and Drug Administration (FDA), means a vitamin or supplement must be in excess of 99 percent purity and contain no binders, fillers, dyes, or unknown substances. Many people complain because these companies are more expensive. But, those companies put their supplements through such rigorous testing that it's often comparable to what the FDA puts pharmaceutical companies through. In some instances, the testing is even above and beyond that of the FDA for purity and lack of radiation.

With nutraceuticals, you get what you pay for—but you are worth it. You only have one body and certainly, if you are taking a supplement, you want to be sure that you are taking what you *think* you are taking. There are certifications for pharmaceutical-grade quality vitamins and minerals and supplements.

We want patients to know that there are certain vitamins that have certification credentials. Look on the bottle and you will find the grade qualities. These vitamins have been researched; their sources are usually organic food sources or whole food sources and they are nonirradiated.

For example, much of the fish oil supplements on the market are available in a gel capsule. The manufacturer must heat that gel capsule to shape it. This heating process *denatures the fish oil,* and the oil will no longer do the same thing inside your body as a cold-pressed fish oil.

Your choice of supplement brand should be influenced by knowing:

- Ingredients in the supplement
- What process is used to make them
- The impact ingredients and processes have on your body

Nutrient Dense and Toxin-Free

Knowing the ingredients applies to food as well as to nutraceuticals. The closer to the source that a food is, the safer you are. Pick single-ingredient foods that are as close to their natural form as possible. The more organic you eat, the less your toxic burden.

Poor food choices can cripple your health. You have probably heard the saying: *garbage in, garbage out.* Think about the packaged foods in your grocery store: foods that are shipped thousands of miles and processed until they're unrecognizable from their origins are devoid of natural vitamins and minerals. If you choose foods like this, you most likely have become nutrient deficient.

Toxins are a whole other issue. Food needs to be tested to have certainty that it is toxin-free. You must make sure that your foods aren't grown in soil that over the years has been exposed to lead, arsenic, and toxic dumping.

With organic foods, you have a better chance of having fewer of those bad things in your food. There's no 100 percent guarantee that organic food growers have been able to keep everything out because our soil is corrupted. Even though we don't have pristine soil, organic growers are required to pass qualifications to become certified, so you can be assured that toxin levels are a lot lower on organic farms.

Choosing non-GMO food is also better. When food is genetically modified, it has been changed from a natural state in which the human body over thousands, or hundreds of thousands of years, has learned to recognize and absorb nutrients from it. When food has been genetically modified and different ingredients are added on a molecular level, your body doesn't quite know how to sort that out and get the nutrients from that food.

Buying from your local farmers, as long as they have healthy farming practices, will help your nutrients to be denser. Many farmers are moving away from organic certification because it is so expensive. Talk to them and become informed—just because they're not certified organic does not mean they are not responsible farmers invested in creating healthy food.

Ask local farmers:

- Do they spray herbicides, insecticides, or fungicides, and if so, are the sprays nontoxic?

- Do they use natural or synthetic fertilizers?

- If you're buying animal products, what do they feed their animals?

Farmers' markets are becoming very popular now, and there are many farmers who are more aware that people are wanting foods that are closer to the source.

One way to get nutrient-dense food is by growing it in your own back yard, or even on your stoop in large pots. More people are also growing their own foods in little six-by-six-foot vegetable gardens. Entering your zip code into the website scorecard.org will provide interesting information about the top chemical polluters in your area, as well as the top chemicals being released. This information will give you an indication what toxic burden might be in your soil. You can also get your soil tested by your cooperative extension office to learn what amendments you might need or if there's anything unsafe in the soil.

CHAPTER THREE

Live Well and Feel Well

The food you eat can either be the safest & most powerful form of Medicine . . . or the slowest form of poison.
~Ann Wigmore

AGING: YOU DON'T HAVE TO FEEL BAD

There are generally five developmental phases in life, called *life stages:*

1. Infancy
2. Childhood
3. Adolescence
4. Adulthood
5. Old age

Each has its own biological, psychological, and social characteristics through which individuals pass during their lives. We want to change that paradigm and help everyone realize that feeling bad is not a condition to be expected.

Unfortunately, our society has cultivated the expectation that it is natural to feel worse as one ages. In many other countries, people are vibrant as long as they live, even into advanced elderly years.

Chronic Pain and Fatigue Are Not Normal

Chronic pain has received a great deal of attention lately, primarily due to all the news about opioid addiction. Opioid pharmaceuticals are easily prescribed to address chronic pain. Unfortunately, it isn't practitioners alone who think opioids are a good solution. Often, insurance companies also tell the medical community that opioids are the cheapest stuff around, so that's what they can prescribe.

You need to realize that it is not mandatory that you suffer. According to the Institute of Medicine (IOM), about 100 million Americans suffer from chronic pain, which is a greater number than diabetes, heart disease, and cancer, combined. Chronic pain is a leading cause of disability among Americans. And, of course, when you are in chronic pain, you have decreased overall enjoyment of life and an increased risk of depression. The IOM also notes that this issue is estimated to cost $600 billion a year in medical treatments.

There are many triggers of chronic pain that people do not realize, such as:

- Emotional trauma
- Poor sleep
- Leaky gut
- Inflammatory foods
- Magnesium deficiency
- Chronic bacterial infections, like Lyme disease

Many natural remedies can make a major difference in pain:

- Lifestyle modifications
- Dietary strategies
- Herbal remedies

Therapies addressing these conditions include:

- Chiropractic
- Physical therapy
- Proper posture
- Massage
- Acupuncture

Fatigue is treated essentially the same as pain. They frequently go hand in hand. Chronic pain and fatigue can have a specific cause, such as Lyme disease or a virus. You want to get to the root cause of pain or fatigue because you can target your treatment better once you've found the reasons for them.

Chronic Diseases Should Not Be Expected

The first major cause of chronic disease is the *standard American diet*. Processed foods have too little fiber, too few micronutrients, and too few omega-3s. The processed or prepared food that people typically eat is laden with sweeteners, especially high fructose corn syrup, which causes high insulin levels. According to the American Heart Association, in 1812, the average American consumed 45 grams of sugar every five days, which is approximately the amount of sugar in a 12 ounce can of today's soda. As of five years ago, the average American consumes 765 grams of sugar every five days, seventeen times as much as our ancestors. Trans fats have been added to our food only in this century. Trans fats overload the mitochondria, which provide energy for the cells, according to studies conducted by the National Institutes of Health.

Another major concern, as we've mentioned before, is toxins in the environment, such as organic pollutants, heavy metals, and other infections. When a toxic burden overwhelms the body's ability to detoxify and heal itself, a chronic disease can arise.

The Weston A. Price Foundation (WestonAPrice.org) evolved from the findings of Dr. Weston Price. He was a dentist in the early twentieth century who searched for the causes of dental decay and physical degeneration he observed in his patients. He decided to travel the world and study isolated human groups. Dr. Price expected to find their health in horrible condition.

Instead, he found beautiful, straight teeth, free from decay, and bodies resistant to disease. Good health was typical of the primitive cultures, fed with their traditional diets rich in essential nutrients. Based on these findings, the organization formed by Dr. Price emphasized whole, nutrient-dense foods.

Through this example, we can see diet makes a huge difference in health. Diet is the foundation of everything.

Memory Loss Is Not Normal

Memory loss is sometimes caused by similar processes of degradation and lesions in the brain that all Alzheimer's patients have. Our culture tends to expect some memory loss with aging, even playfully referring to lapses in memory as *senior moments*. The same lifestyle choices that will lower your risk of diabetes will also help improve your chance of keeping your mind intact. Diet and exercise go hand in hand to form your primary defense against disease, including all brain disorders.

Age is the greatest risk factor for Alzheimer's and dementia, but the insulin resistance of diabetes significantly increases your risk. You do not need to increase sugar and carbs; the brain does not run like that. A diet rich in vegetables and fats is gaining significant credibility as a preventative of memory loss. Vegetables have major anti-oxidants and protect from oxidative stress, and the brain uses fat as its major source of food. The American diet has become fat deficient.

Exercise encourages the brain to run at its optimal capacity. According to Harvard Health Publishing, exercise helps memory and thinking through both direct and indirect means. Benefits of exercise come directly from its ability to reduce insulin resistance, reduce inflammation, and stimulate the release of growth factors—chemicals in the brain that affect the health of brain cells, the growth of new blood vessels in the brain, and even the abundance and survival of new brain cells.

Indirectly, exercise improves mood and sleep, and reduces stress and anxiety. Problems in these areas frequently cause or contribute to cognitive impairment.

Alzheimer's is sometimes called *type 3 diabetes* by some experts.

The four major memory enemies are:

1. Sugar, especially fructose
2. Grains
3. Aspartame
4. Soy

There are multiple influences on memory loss. Toxic exposures accumulate over the years; unfortunately, we now live in a very toxic world.

Certain occupations, as well as some hobbies, increase your risk for toxic substances, such as:

- Arsenic
- Lead
- Organophosphates
- Cadmium
- Mercury

While some changes may not be reversible, others are. If we can discover the cause and remove the offending agent, there may be improvement in cognitive function.

What else can we do to support brain health?

Significant components of optimum brain function include vitamin D and omega-3 fatty acids, especially DHA, predominantly found in cold water, fatty fish, such as salmon. Our portion sizes are also a problem—as a nation, we simply eat too much. You can consider whether you need to limit how much you eat in a day. Another beneficial step is to limit your intake of soy, since it is one of the largest GMO crops in the U.S. Unfermented soy, such as tofu, is not a healthy food, despite its reputation. Fermented soy is far more usable by our bodies. Sources include nato and tempeh.

HOW DO YOU ACCOMPLISH AGING WELL?

You need to be aware—practicing self-awareness and introspection—about what you are doing with your life. Today, with the extreme stresses we are under, many people run on the treadmill of life. Before they know it, they are looking back with regrets about what they could have and should have done.

Many patients come to us with a misconception that how their parents aged is how they are going to age. They feel if their parents have chronic disease, they are going to develop chronic disease. We want them to know that *chronic disease is not a normal part of aging*. You can change the genetic cards dealt you at birth. You can move them around and make them in your favor—if you know how to do the correct thing. Genetics constitutes about 5 percent of disease risk and the other 95 percent is due to lifestyle choices and environmental exposures.

It is difficult to discern what of the abundantly available information is merely fad and what information is reliable. Knowing the difference between the two is essential to accomplishing the goal of aging well.

Embrace and Enjoy the Phases of Life

The greatest thief of enjoyment in the various phases of life is stress. Many Americans report being under extreme stress, and many experts believe that stress can contribute to chronic disease. When people don't have effective stress management techniques, they choose unhealthy coping strategies to deal with stress, such as soothing the self by watching TV, drinking alcohol, or eating junk food.

Some people have genetic or epigenetic processes that cause personality traits associated with excessive worry. These can be helped through nutrients and nutraceutical treatments. Also, stress management techniques, such as meditation, can help relieve the effects of stress. By embracing each phase of your life, you can be more fulfilled and happy.

Dr. Geszler has a personal reflection on the phase of women's lives that is menopause:

My mother started having problems with her health at age fifty. She was a worrier; she used to become anxious and worried about many things. After menopause, she was in chronic pain. Her health deteriorated and she was miserable. She lived forty years beyond menopause and didn't seem very happy after it. Forty years is a very long time, and my memory of her was of her misery. My mother could not embrace that phase or subsequent phases.

I decided not to live like that. I embraced a totally different life, taking charge of my health—exercising, eating well, and enjoying each day. I am now sixty-five, and proud of it, largely because I wear it well.

> *It is encouraging for people to note that it is difficult to tell my age.*

Being proactive and choosing a healthy lifestyle early on makes a difference. We can look to our parents to help decide how we want to continue living as adults.

Do you want to take the same path, or a different one?

We can elect to take the path to become more serious about nutrition and exercise and head in the direction toward a healthier life.

Be Proactive in Your Younger Years

Dr. Pam Smith, our fellowship director in anti-aging, regenerative, and functional medicine, once said, "Anti-aging begins at birth."

It is never too early to examine your health on various levels. It is easier to prevent disease than to reverse it. Some things can be reversed, but in many cases, once you've done the damage, the damage is done. The younger you are when you embrace a healthier lifestyle, the better your chances of preventing chronic disease and remaining vibrant through your life.

Strategies to remember:

- Eat right—consume a variety of whole foods.
- Sleep right—aim for at least seven hours of sleep a night.
- Exercise right—at least move regularly throughout the day.

Also, walk barefoot to ground yourself to Earth. Emerging research published in the *Journal of Environmental and Public Health* shows electrons from the soil have antioxidant effects that can protect your body from inflammation. Being in direct contact with the earth grounds your body and induces physiological change that promotes optimal health. There's a lot to be said for walking barefoot in the park.

A sedentary lifestyle is a major contributor to chronic disease and disability. Get plenty of fresh air and sunshine. Never have we, as a species, spent so much time indoors, exposed to toxic chemicals in the air, EMFs (electromagnetic fields), and suffering from severe vitamin D deficiency. There is nothing more important than your health, it should be your most precious valuable—that which you value most in your life.

Attitude Is Everything

> *Happiness resides not in possessions and not in gold;*
> *happiness grows in the soul.*
> ~ Democritus

> *If you have health you probably will be happy.*
> *And if you have health and happiness*
> *you have all the wealth you need,*
> *even if it is not all you want.*
> ~ Elbert Hubbard

> *Learn to forgive successfully and completely.*
> *If you want health, wealth, and happiness,*
> *you can't afford the luxury of lugging around all those*
> *unforgiving unforgotten past events. Let them go.*
> ~ Peter McWilliams

Happiness often resides in material possessions for a lot people. Striving for the best car, best house, best clothes, or best job is about as beneficial as the daily blast of bravado you get from Facebook.

Spiritual attitude is everything. You must look inside and examine your spiritual self. Some people use religion to guide them, but, it doesn't matter how you find that health, happiness, and peacefulness within; it really goes a long way to make you an overall healthy, happy person.

Happiness is directly linked to health. Most people who are truly happy don't have many health problems. People who are miserable or in a bad situation—maybe they are in a job they hate but stay because they make a lot of money—they are not happy, and, therefore, their health suffers tremendously.

DOING THE THINGS YOU WANT TO DO

A *Forbes* magazine article discussed how happiness comes from choosing to be happy with whatever you do, as well as strengthening your closest relationships and caring for yourself physically, emotionally, and financially.[1]

Many people get on a treadmill in life:

1. They graduate from high school.
2. They graduate from college.
3. They fall in love and get married.
4. They start a family.

But, some people simply don't fit in that mold.

What is happiness *to you?*

Imagine what kind of life you would like to have and try to pick the things that make you happy.

1   Bradt, George. "The Secret of Happiness Revealed by Harvard Study." Forbes. 5/27/15. forbes.com

Don't Rank Possessions Over Health and Happiness

The *Forbes* article reports that, in 2010, researchers surveyed Harvard graduates from the class of 1980 and concluded that happiness among these graduates accrued from three things:

1. Doing good for others—cherishing their most important relationships and being a contribution to their community.

2. Doing things that they are good at—doing more of what they are good at and less of what they are not good at.

3. Doing things which are good for themselves—taking care of their health and well-being and maintaining their work/life balance.

Achieve Balance in Your Life

We recently read a study conducted by professors of psychology at the University of Rochester that revealed when people's goals were extrinsic—wealth, fame, personal image—they were less happy than those whose goals were intrinsic, such as meaningful relationships, health, and personal growth.[2] When one focuses on the extrinsic, materialistic things, it's

2   University of Rochester. "Achieving Fame, Wealth and Beauty Are Psychological Dead Ends, Study Says." *ScienceDaily*, 19 May 2009.

impossible to have a good life-balance because relationships, health, and personal growth will get ignored.

Enjoy Things in Front of You

When we see patients in their older years, the biggest regret they usually have is they didn't take care of themselves. They regret that now because of their disease. They're not able to enjoy their grandchildren and their life accomplishments. Often, we see that when people retire it is almost like they begin to die.

In life, it is very important to find balance, so work hard and accomplish your goals, but keep an endgame you can be happy with. *You want to be able enjoy what you've accomplished.* Don't work yourself so hard to accomplish your goals that you make yourself sick.

Find a balance in your day that allows you to build the life you want, but also live in a healthy way. Stay mindful that you want to and can enjoy your retirement, time with grandchildren, or whatever you want to do as you get older. Cynthia has grandkids, and she enjoys them completely because they are the most wonderful children on the Earth!

Again, don't just focus on the end goal of retirement, but enjoy each step along the way:

- Enjoy your children and all steps and phases they go through.

- Enjoy the people around you and cherish those relationships.

- Show appreciation for the people around you.

- Show how much you care about them.

Keep your friends. So many people as they get older start losing friends through death or relocation. Some people don't have family. There are some who have not married and they don't have children, or for some reason something has happened with the relationship. It's important to keep social connections because your friends are the ones who are going to carry you through and help to balance your life.

The social interactions that come with having friends keeps your mind healthy. You want to surround yourself with people who enrich you and make you a better person in different ways. They don't have to be exactly like you, and it is actually better to find people who are different from you because they will stimulate you to think differently.

> *. . . My wife is able to work and enjoy life because of the things you have helped her deal with. Her mother, sister, and grandmother all have suffered and their quality of life diminished. So thankful to you for making it possible for my wife to feel good about life and enjoy it with me. You really are a blessing to us.*
>
> ~ T. and B.

CHAPTER FOUR

Emotional Health
Is a Critical Element

Take rest; a field that has rested gives a bountiful crop.
~ Ovid

NEGATIVE EMOTIONS CAN BOYCOTT YOUR OVERALL HEALTH

No one can truly be well without dealing with their emotional health and eliminating negative emotions.

Negative Emotions Cause Physiological Stress

We all know stress can come from many sources in life, for example:

- Relationships
- Jobs
- Health
- Commitments

Anyone who does not get enough rest and relaxation, who drives themselves constantly, who is never satisfied, or who becomes the perfectionist under constant pressure without an outlet for emotional release, is subject to the subsequent ill effects of stress. Someone who feels trapped or helpless, overwhelmed by repeated or continual difficulties, or who has experienced severe or chronic emotional or physical trauma or illness is also at risk of suffering the ill effects of stress.

The ill effects of stress are usually due to excess *cortisol,* which becomes elevated by both physical and emotional stress. The body is not designed for prolonged, extreme, and unlimited stress.

Chronically elevated cortisol causes deleterious health effects, such as:

- Damage to brain cells
- Elevated blood sugars
- Increased pulse
- Elevated blood pressure
- Compromised reproductive function
- Reduced thyroid function
- Reduced circulating thyroid hormone

The elevated cortisol from prolonged stress can also dampen your immune response, which can cause multiple illnesses. It wreaks havoc with your intestinal tract and your digestive system. Elevated cortisol causes sleeplessness because your brain is more aware, or hypervigilant. Also, it can suppress your growth hormones, which help repair tissues, so it also can affect your ability to heal—which can affect the way you respond to cancer cells.

Face the Causes of Negative Emotions

Physical symptoms related to unresolved trauma include:

- Eating disturbances
- Sleep disturbances
- Sexual disturbances
- Low energy
- Chronic, unexplained pain

Emotional symptoms can be:

- Depression
- Anxiety
- Fearfulness
- Panic attacks

Cognitive symptoms can be:

- Memory lapses
- ADD/ADHD symptoms
- Difficulties with decision making

The first step in our approach to healing is expressed by this quote of Albert Ellis:

*The best years of your life are ones in which
you decide your problems are your own.
You do not blame them on your mother,
the ecology, or the president.
You realize that you control your own destiny.*

Be Willing to Change

We think making lists of pros and cons of various problems is helpful. One approach is to make a list of all the things that help your health and then a list of all the things that harm your health and well-being. So, things that help health are enjoyable things that bring love to life, even if you have not done them for a while. Things that would harm your health could include negative physical and emotional patterns, attitudes, work, relationship and family situations, and eating and drinking patterns.

When you find yourself in detrimental situations, you must decide on one of three actions:

1. Change the situation.
2. Change yourself.
3. Leave the situation.

*Things turn out best for people
who make the best of the way things turn out.*
~ John Wooden

HOW TO MANAGE STRESS

If you don't manage your stressors, you will not achieve health; they can simply tear you down. First, you must be able to recognize what is causing your stress. If you can't recognize what the stress is, you can't manage it. Next, it is important to work with your functional medicine doctor, and probably a counselor or a therapist, to help you get down to the nitty-gritty of what's going on with your emotional, as well as physical, health.

Recognize the Signs of Stress in Your Body

Life for many people has become such a rat race that stress is prevalent and accepted as a way of life. Many people don't recognize stress until it becomes catastrophic. Everybody varies in how much stress they can handle, and some of that ability is inherited. Much depends on the lifestyle habits you've developed.

There are subtle signs to recognize negative stress in your body, such as:

- A knot in your stomach
- Tightening of muscles in your neck or elsewhere
- Stress eating
- Insomnia
- Needing stimulants to function
- Physical and emotional exhaustion

- Loss of perspective
- Lack of connection with work
- Depression

Burnout often results from long-term, excessive stress. To recover from stress or burnout, the best strategy is a combination of diet, exercise, and mindfulness with stress reduction.

Consider any or of a combination of the following:

- A healthy diet that is nutrient dense and whole-food based

- Making time for your social network, family, spirituality, or meditation

- Exercise to help lower cortisol—as long as it is not excessive exercise

Many people think physical manifestations—such as anxiety, feeling a knot in their stomach, or feeling like they have gastric problems—must all be related to something physical. But, these symptoms can also be related to your mental health. Unresolved issues, such as trauma or stress, are often associated with symptoms, like depression, anxiety, and sleep issues.

With unresolved trauma or stress, symptoms can include:

- Nightmares
- Flashbacks
- Addiction problems

Many people self-medicate with alcohol or street drugs because they are trying to hide stress or problems, and they don't recognize these signs of increased stress and past trauma.

Consult a Stress-Management Expert

Many people have difficulty being introspective. But, introspection is necessary when choosing solutions to your own stress. Sometimes, family, social circles, or church can offer all the support one may need to get through stress. But, sometimes not. When you are not able to figure out how to manage your stress, seeing someone who specializes in that area is a good idea.

Traditionally, we often think of psychiatrists and psychologists as stress management experts. For many people, it may be intimidating to need a psychiatric diagnosis to see a specialist.

Today there are many other options to help people deal with stress, such as:

- Energy medical practitioners, who can facilitate emotional and physical relief

- Online tutorials for *emotional freedom techniques* (EFT), such as meridian tapping therapy

- Relaxation apps available for the computer, phone, or tablet

These options can be very useful to deal with ongoing stress, and it's all a matter of degree. Some people have a small amount of stress and they can deal with it, helping themselves. But, for more emotional issues and deeper trauma, a therapist may be needed. It may be appropriate to have an initial consultation with a medical doctor who can work through the symptoms and give you direction.

Venture Outside Your Comfort Zone

Often, just acknowledging your stressors is enough to pull you out of your comfort zone. Balance is the most important thing that you must attain to live a long life as a whole person. To achieve balance, you need to consider what you do daily.

Who do you interact with daily, and what are your priorities?

There are four components to everyone's life:

- Physical
- Spiritual
- Work
- Relationships

If any one or more is ignored and the balance becomes skewed, then your overall health will suffer. Only with reflection can you evaluate if you are out of balance. This could be a new concept and totally out of your comfort zone. However, as you develop mindful awareness of all aspects of your life, you can develop strategies for dealing with stressors and imbalances.

DEALING WITH UNRESOLVED TRAUMA

It can be difficult to recognize past trauma. Some people suffer unknowingly from past trauma. Even though they don't remember the past trauma, it negatively impacts their daily life.

You can block out the trauma cognitively yet still experience the physical effects from it. It may take courage and faith to face your past, examine your life, and face people who have caused you pain. Healing your past traumatic experiences help you create a joyful, healthy present moment, and open the doors to the life you want for yourself. Emotional healing will create positive physical changes in your body.

Resurfacing Events Affect Your Health

Unresolved trauma can affect your habits and outlook on life. It can be devastating in your life because, as mentioned before, it can trigger physical pain, addictive behavior, difficulty with relationships, and can cause chronic illness due to abnormal cortisol level. Unresolved trauma may lead to physical, emotional, and mental illness.

It is important to pay attention to your signs and symptoms and be willing to explore these with your medical doctor or counselor. Because you may not be aware of the trauma, it is also important to explore this as a part of illness that may not be resolved by other methods. There are many patients who see their family doctor and have labs and are treated but are told all is normal. Many physical illnesses are actually manifestations of psychological issues.

When you are told everything looks normal, but you haven't regained your health, it is time to explore options of treatment that consider unresolved trauma.

Traumatic events you may not realize can affect you can include:

- Natural disasters
- Physical assaults
- Serious accidents
- Witnessing horrific events
- Serious illnesses
- Falls or injuries
- Birth trauma
- Surgery—especially emergency surgery early in life

Explore Your Emotional Past

If your primary healthcare provider tells you everything is fine but you still feel unwell, you may then decide to consult a functional medicine doctor. They will probably explore your thyroid, gut health, and your adrenals. A functional medicine doctor will dig deeper into your symptoms, probably more than anyone else has in the past.

Yet, you may still have all the signs and symptoms you originally experienced. Or, perhaps you have had a slight improvement, but you and your functional medicine doctor don't feel you have progressed as far as you should. This is the time to consider unresolved emotional trauma may be causing some of your physical symptoms.

When you come to this point, you must look at the signs and symptoms again. It may be necessary to delve into the past and uncomfortable memories that could be triggering your physical pain.

If you recognize any of these signs and they are not resolved with medical treatment, then ask yourself if it is time to talk to a therapist or a counselor:

- Sleep issues
- Fatigue
- Avoidance

Recognition of a problem is the first basic step to healing. Much of this came to light in the 1990s with Adverse Childhood Experiences (ACE) studies. A study of 17,000 patients conducted by researchers at the Center for Disease Control and Kaiser Permanente in Southern California assessed the link between emotional experiences and adult health and were able to provide very compelling evidence that childhood trauma and instability impact health outcomes. The participants were asked about ten forms of personal abuse or dysfunctional family behavior before the age of eighteen. For additional information, refer to acestoohigh. com/got-your-ace-score.

The results were stunning. More than half of the participants had an adverse childhood experiences. Of those who did, they were forty to fifty times more likely to have an adverse health condition in adulthood.

After exploring standard medical treatments, ask yourself:

Have I really improved, or is something holding me back from full recovery?

Am I having feelings of being emotionally drained, or just feeling dead inside?

If the answer to those questions is *yes,* then it is time to seek counseling from an expert.

Let Go, Accept, or Resolve the Trauma

Remember, you have options:

- Seek the help of a therapist or a counselor.
- Consult an energy practitioner.
- Use apps available for your phone, tablet, or computer.

You may have stress or past trauma that is affecting you physically but trying to resolve the symptoms medically will not result in resolution. Often, once the cause is recognized, it is a relief to know there is a path to wellness. Learning techniques is only the first step on your journey to healing, and it is important to develop the technique that works for you.

Our Personal Technique

At night, our minds wonder about the stresses of the day and what we expect to face tomorrow. We could take medication to help us fall asleep, but we discovered a meditation app for our smartphones which works well for each of us. Before turning in for the night, we might listen to it for five to ten minutes. This app teaches us how to be mindful, accept the things we can't change, and look at the world with more appreciation.

Listening to the lessons from the app helps us to reflect on how we approach each day. It puts our mind at rest and helps us concentrate on the things we need most—which is restorative sleep. This works for us, but it may not work for you.

You must explore on your own, using the many resources available, to discover what helps you to be mindful. *Mindfulness* is a mental practice of focusing one's awareness on the present moment while calmly acknowledging and accepting one's feelings, thoughts, and bodily sensations. You first reframe your perspective by observing physical sensations, such as where you feel your body making contact with your seat or the floor, your breath expanding ribs and belly, and what you can hear around you. This helps ground you in the moment, free from emotional concern of what was or what will be. From this neutral place, you can examine what is causing you stress, and acknowledge and accept it without trying to change it. Once you see what is causing you stress, you reframe it—you change the mental context of it.

Once you learn to accept the feelings you have within—whether it's anger, frustration, unfairness, or sadness—you can change the way you think of the problem and reframe it. You can regard what has caused you stress in a different way. This is a mindfulness practice, and it helps you view your emotions differently, so you can accept them and yourself.

The results of mindfulness are:

- Better sleep and restfulness
- Healthier body

Mindfulness takes practice; it is not a technique that comes naturally to us. We must teach our mind to look at problems in a different way.

The smartphone app we elected to use each night gives us kudos on how many sessions we each have explored. We get positive reinforcement and have a feeling of making progress but appreciate the fact that one or two sessions does not make us experts. We are willing to explore different methods and techniques. We often remind ourselves of the need to keep our minds open, be willing to learn, and let go.

You must accept the trauma from your past to resolve it or accept it. If you have lived through traumatic events that continue to affect you, emotionally letting go will be liberating for your future mental and physical health. Both physical and mental stressors interact, and both must be addressed for complete health.

Remember:

- A poor diet reduces your body's ability to respond to stress.

- The basic principle of healing is to remove health-limiting factors, such as junk foods, drugs, alcohol, excess caffeine, and stimulants.

To address emotional issues, explore what is draining you emotionally and learn to let go. If the stress is ongoing, learn to stand up for yourself.

CHAPTER FIVE

Why Exercise Is Important

A man's health can be judged by which
he takes two at a time—pills or stairs.
~ Joan Welsh

EVERYONE CAN EXERCISE

As society has changed, physical labor is no longer a part of most peoples' lives. Everyday conveniences, such as washing machines, vacuum cleaners, snowblowers, lawnmowers, and remote controls, have severely restricted our movement. Unless you are a construction worker or someone in an intensely physical job, you need exercise.

The benefits of exercise are:

- Helps prevent disease
- Keeps your mind sharp
- Prevents osteoporosis
- Prevents depression
- Increases your balance and strength

There's No Age Limit for Exercise

Numerous studies sponsored by the National Institutes of Health (NIH), several of which have been publicized in the journal *Biogerontology* in the past decade, have evaluated the use of exercise for the elderly and frail.[3] Regular physical activity has been determined to help improve physical and mental functions, as well as reverse some effects of chronic disease to keep older people mobile and independent. Exercise has been shown to increase gait speed, balance, and improve the activities performed in daily living. Studies have also determined that elderly people with cardiovascular disease, pulmonary disease, or arthritis all benefit from exercise.

One of our patients, in her seventies, came to us after she went on a vacation with her family and realized she was unable to keep up with them. She was so fatigued she had to stop frequently and rest. She was fed up with feeling this way. She came to our wellness program and found out how important exercise is to feeling healthy. She got a personal trainer, started lifting weights, and is now able to vacation and do all the activities she could not do before.

Data suggest a correlation between improved muscular strength and balance and positive changes in psychological functioning.

Physical activity helps:

---

3   *Biogerontology*. 2016; 17: 567–580.

- Increase energy
- Cultivate a positive mood
- Lessen insomnia

Regular exercise helps you look and feel better, and it's just as beneficial in your seventies as in your twenties. *You are never too old to start.* Studies show that people who start exercise later in life gain better physical and mental improvement than their younger counterparts.[4]

Exercise is the number-one contributor to longevity. It helps shed excess weight and maintain healthy weight. Exercise reduces chronic pain and disease, and increases mobility, flexibility, balance, quality sleep, boosts mood, and helps with self-control. You can begin maintenance exercise at any age. Although it can be a challenge because starting doesn't get easier as you get older; it is much *more beneficial* for you as you get older.

There Is an Exercise for You

When we talk to people about exercise, we divide it up into four categories:

1. Endurance
2. Strength
3. Balance
4. Flexibility

---

4   *Comprehensive Physiology.* 2013 Jan; 3(1): 403–428.

Anyone at any level can pick different exercises for each of these components.

1. **Endurance exercises** increase your breathing and heart rate. Examples include brisk walking, swimming, and hiking. Building your endurance makes everyday activities, such as mowing the lawn or climbing stairs, easier. And, besides getting back to raking the yard and bagging weeds, you will be able to do more enjoyable activities like keeping up with your grandchildren and dancing at a wedding.

2. **Strength exercises** need to include a variety of exercises. They can be lifting weights or pulling against resistance bands, and will help with simple daily activities, such as: lifting luggage into an overhead bin on a plane, picking up bags of mulch in the garden, and carrying groceries from your car.

3. **Balance exercises** are critical to help prevent falls, which are very common in the elderly, but they can also occur in younger people. Improved balanced can help assist you in things, such as turning around quickly to face somebody behind you, walking along a gravel path without losing your balance, or standing on tip toes to reach the top shelf.

4. **Flexibility** is achieved through stretching. Staying flexible and limber helps you to keep freedom of movement, which in turn helps your daily activities,

such as bending over to tie your shoes, looking over your shoulder when backing up in the car, and stretching to clean hard to reach places of your home.

Build a balanced exercise plan that includes varied activities:

- Walking
- Jogging
- Dancing
- Weight lifting

Remember that daily activities, such as housecleaning, are also exercise. Mix it up. Do strength and power training like weight lifting, along with balance and flexibility training, such as yoga, qigong, or tai chi.

Get Out of That Chair!

When thinking about your health, you want to work on your mindset. Exercise is an essential element of your optimal health, every bit as important as nutrients. But, whatever you do, do not consider exercise as an offset to an unhealthy diet.

Health benefits of regular exercise include:

- Strengthening your immune system
- Lowering your cancer rate
- Decreasing your insulin
- Lowering your diabetes risk
- Reducing damage from free radicals

- Increasing your productivity
- Slowing your aging by as much as ten years
- Improving your memory

If establishing a routine of movement or exercise is a big change, or you have pre-existing conditions, you could be adversely affected by doing too much too fast. So, before you get out of the chair and start to exercise, the first thing you need to do is get medical clearance. Discuss with your doctor what exercises you can do safely. Also, consider your ongoing health problems and whether you need to adjust the timing or any types of exercise that you do.

Listen to your body. You *should not* hurt or feel lousy after you exercise. If you experience any shortness of breath, chest pain, or any type of intense pain, you should stop immediately and call your doctor. If a joint becomes red or swollen, then you need to stop, rest, and take care of it—then, later restart the program. *The key is to start slowly and build steadily.* Any type of injury will, of course, slow you down, but take good care of yourself so you can continue.

As you exercise, remember these ideas:

- Practice mindfulness for your exercise routine.
- Commit to an exercise schedule so it becomes habit.
- Experiment with mindfulness instead of zoning out.
- Focus during your exercise.

- Notice how your body feels as you move to get a rhythm.
- Notice how your muscles feel as you are exercising.

HOW TO PICK THE CORRECT EXERCISE

There is not one exercise that's right for everyone, and one exercise alone cannot do it all for you. You must pick from different categories and see what your goals are according to the phase of life you are in. Everyone has societal and life commitments, which can limit your time for exercise, but you must not use it as an excuse to not exercise. It is important to reserve at least a couple hours per week for exercise in your schedule.

Start at Beginning Levels

There are many reasons you will have decided it is time to start an exercise program, for example, your doctor may have told you to do so for your health, or someone may have given you a gift membership to a gym.

Whatever the reason, you may not be sure how to begin. Well, rest assured there is no magic formula. Just remember: the most important reason you are starting is *for your health*. You want to live a healthier life and reduce your risk of chronic disease and prevent cancer.

But, how do you start and where do you begin?

The best place to start, as the saying goes, is at the beginning. First, decide what level of exercise is appropriate for you—and, if it is truly starting from ground zero, then start out by simply moving. Little increments of exercise will greatly boost your whole well-being. You can choose to walk, garden, bike, or dance. Yard work and household chores also count toward your movement goals.

Starting with five to ten minutes of movement will get you on your way toward a thirty-minute-per-day goal. There are many ways to measure the intensity of your exercise. You can know how hard you are working by measuring your heart rate. There are several apps available to help you figure out what your target rate should be.

As with any new exercise, or change in activity level, please check with your health provider to make sure your heart is healthy enough for physical activity. If you have never exercised, and if you are young and have no physical limitations, you are less likely to hurt yourself. However, as you age, you become more likely to cause injury.

It is important to go slowly. If you decide you want to do yoga, don't go into a power yoga course, but take a beginner's yoga course instead. If you go to a gym, don't just start lifting weights on your own without knowing what you're doing—seek some guidance and help and do light weights, not heavy weights. Always begin slowly and work your way up.

Exercising in this way helps prevent injury, which could be discouraging and interrupt your program.

Seek the Help of an Expert

Thinking about a comprehensive exercise program?

Look at the different types of exercises:

- Endurance exercise can be walking, running, hiking, swimming, elliptical, stationary bike.

  Years ago, it was thought that running and jogging were the way to go. But, then it was discovered that high intensity interval training (HIIT)—or short bursts of activity with intervals of rest in between—improves your fat burning and cardiovascular fitness. HIIT should only be undertaken with guidance because if you have a medical condition, you could cause yourself more problems.

- For strength training, you want to build your strength and maintain muscle mass, increase your metabolic rate, and support your skeleton and joints.

  Many women are afraid that they will bulk up and look manly. And, elderly and even young children may think that strength training is too risky or dangerous. But, science shows that moderate weight lifting may be the best exercise for lifetime function and fitness. Remember, if you have never done it before, you want someone who knows what they are doing to guide you.

- Balance and flexibility exercises include Pilates, yoga, and stretching. These exercises help your abdomen and lower back and go a long way to avoid injury with everyday activities. They keep you limber and help to maintain your range of motion.

  Many people can easily pull muscles in their back with a simple little twist because they are not strengthening their core. Stretching is also often ignored but often helps reduce lower back pain and prevents injuries.

The internet is flush with information. You can use Google to find stretching and basic core exercises. There are numerous home exercises for many of the issues you want to address.

A study in 2017, sponsored by the Iowa State University College of Human Sciences, showed gym membership was related to fourteen times higher odds of meeting weekly physical activity guidelines.[5] Yet, many people with gym memberships never go. So, if you join a gym, *you need to go*. Capitalize on the people who are available at the gym with

5   Schroeder, E. C., et al., "Associations of Health Club Membership with Physical Activity and Cardiovascular Health." *PLoS ONE* 12(1): e0170471. 2017. doi.org/10.1371/journal. pone.0170471

the knowledge that can guide you and help you reach your goals.

There are experts and teachers available in any of these various exercises. This is what they do for a living, so you shouldn't be ashamed to ask them for help and seek their guidance. Remember, none of us was born with this knowledge. Nobody knows how to do yoga from birth. Nobody knows how to stretch from birth. Nobody knows how to run effectively from birth.

Find some people who know more about fitness than you—it is always good to seek guidance and help. If you are not able to afford a gym membership, there are many apps on your phone that can help you connect with personal trainers. Many personal trainers have podcasts and DVDs. You must choose the venue that works out the best for you.

Work Within Your Physical Limitations

If you are severely overweight or disabled, you may not be able to perform all types of exercises. If all you can do is stand and take some deep breaths, begin there. Maybe you can begin with ten minutes of body movement within your own home. If you join a gym, resist comparing yourself to those who look more physically fit and experienced; instead, focus on your needs and your progress. This is not to say you cannot learn from those who are similar in age to you who are physically fit. Note the exercises they do and learn from them.

Again, the internet has resources for balance and coordination exercises, beginners' guides to strength training, and exercises using your own body weight which you can do at home.

What do we mean by start *slowly?*

If you have led a sedentary life up until now, and have a sedentary job, you can start by setting a timer that will alert you every thirty minutes to get up and move. You can walk, run, or jump in place; you can do a few squats, you can stand and stretch, you can even do a little dance or a jig. But the point is to simply start moving. If you are sitting in front of the TV for six hours a day, this can shorten your life span *by five to ten years.*

As you build up to longer periods of movement, you want to start with a five- to ten-minute warm-up. Keep your breath slow and natural. Move slowly and steadily, but gently stretch your legs, your arms, shoulders, and your back. As you stretch, avoid bouncing because this can cause muscle injury.

Specific stretches can be found on the internet, or in classes, or with a trainer. Monitor your pulse rate, or *target heart range,* to track your ability and your fitness.[6] You can use that as a key to discovering whether you're training at a good rate

---

6   Your *target heart rate* is defined as the minimum number of heartbeats in a given amount of time in order to reach the level of exertion necessary for cardiovascular fitness, specific to a person's age, gender, or physical fitness.

for you—something that will burn off extra weight but not endanger your health. When you start, your pulse rate may get very fast, then as you continue to exercise, gradually get slower. You can build your heart rate toward your target.

MORE IS NOT NECESSARILY BETTER

When it applies to any exercise, anything in excess can be detrimental to your health.

Many people think: *Well, if I run a mile, then maybe I should try to run twenty-six miles.*

The more prudent approach is to consider perhaps a 5k, or 10k road race, or half-marathon well before considering a full marathon.

Many people focus on one exercise to the exclusion of all other exercises. To strengthen your entire body, you should lead an active life with a lot of movement as part of a well-balanced exercise strategy—not just one type of exercise along the way. An excessive amount of exercise can have destructive effects on the body.

Simple Movements Lower Your Disease Risk

Obesity is just one side effect of insufficient movement. Inactivity has been linked to multiple diseases and ailments, raising the risk for all ill health significantly, such as with Alzheimer's and depression. Being sedentary for long periods during the day seems to accelerate aging at the cellular level.

Some call sitting the *new smoking*. Each cigarette reduces your life by eleven minutes, whereas Dr. James Levine, co-director of the Obesity Initiative for Mayo Clinic/Arizona State University, and author of the book *Get Up! Why Your Chair Is Killing You and What You Can Do About It*, found that for every hour that you sit, your life shortens by two hours. And your ability to get up from a sitting position on the floor to a standing position is associated with an increased risk of death within the next six years, if you are unable to do so.[7]

Sedentary lifestyle is a serious risk in our society, but simple movements can lower your risk of disease. Lack of exercise has been shown to be a serious health risk, especially for cardiovascular disease as well as other diseases.

Disease processes affected by inactivity include:

- Diabetes
- Coronary artery disease
- Obesity
- Depression
- Anxiety
- Decreased bone density

---

7   Blog interview by Dr. Joseph Mercola with James A. Levine. 9/28/2014. articles.mercola.com/sites/articles/archive/2014/09/28/dangers-prolonged-sitting.aspx

- Certain cancers

The more sedentary you are, the weaker your bones become. Without muscle tone, your mobility starts to suffer. Weakness and brittle bones together are a recipe for falls and crippling disability. According to the World Health Organization, 60 to 85 percent of the population does not engage in enough activity.[8] Globally, it is the fourth-leading cause of mortality.

Thirty minutes of daily exercise cannot counter the effects of a sedentary lifestyle the rest of the day. So, it is recommended that you have a goal of 10,000 steps, or five miles, per day. In a 2005 *Science* magazine article, Dr. Levine labeled a sedentary lifestyle, "the disease of our time."

If you are older, falls can impact the activities of your daily living. There are thousands of deaths attributed yearly due to lack of exercising, or lack of physical activity. Statistically, most people reduce activity as they age and women reduce their activity more than men.[9]

Start Slowly and Gradually Increase

Up to 50 percent of people who start a new exercise program will stop within six months. In our experience, so many people come to the gym and get all gung ho, just to be so sore

---

8   World Health Organization News Release. 4/4/2002. who.int/mediacentre/news/releases/release23/en
9   McPhee, James. "Physical Activity in Older age: Perspective for Healthy Aging and Frailty." *Biogerontology*. March 2, 2016.

the next day they can barely get out of bed. But, the secret to maintaining an exercise program long term is to avoid overexertion early in the game. You should feel comfortable with your level of activity before you move on to the next one. Your exercise level should not cause you to feel miserable the next day.

Getting a fitness tracker is also a great idea to help push you to move and try to get in those 10,000 steps a day. Some recommendations, including those from government agencies, say an individual needs a minimum of 150 minutes of moderate exercise per week. For adults, that's at least two-and-half hours of moderate aerobic activity that works all major muscle groups and muscle strengthening activities on two or more days per week. This recommendation for exercise guidelines comes directly from the Department of Health and Human Services.

Then, for even greater health benefits, you should do five hours of moderate aerobic exercise and muscle strengthening activities divided into sessions no longer than one hour. Changing from a sedentary lifestyle to an active lifestyle takes a specific action plan. Researchers found people were more successful in sustaining their new lifestyle when they tracked their activity.

There are several ways to do this:

1. You can write it down, the old-fashioned way, or you can find free apps for your phone, or you can buy an electronic fitness tracker.

2. Set your specific goals. At first it can be as simple as 10,000 steps or five miles of activity per day.

Cynthia Phillips previously worked with a patient, "Vivian", who led a sedentary life and had a history of diabetes. When Vivian came to her initial appointment, she commented to Ms. Phillips that she could not understand why she was having such a hard time losing weight and felt so bad.

Ms. Phillips suggested Vivian purchase a Fitbit tracker to monitor the number of steps she took daily. When Vivian came back, she reported that she realized she had only been moving 800 steps per day. So, during the next three months, Vivian increased her activity. When Vivian returned after those three months, she had gotten up to her 10,000 steps a day, had lost ten pounds, was going out with her friends, was feeling much better, and had a lot more activity in her life.

Shorter Duration of Intense Exercise Is More Effective Than Longer

You may feel overwhelmed if you think you need to exercise for a long time. Many people focus only on cardiovascular fitness or heavy weight lifting instead of looking at a balanced approach. It's been shown that if you exercise for more than sixty minutes, that you use up your body's glycogen and you start stimulating cortisol.[10]

Cortisol is the stress hormone. Its effects are meant to be short-lived for quick stress, but when you prolong the stress, your muscle starts to break down. When you overexercise and produce more cortisol, you're actually working against your goal. Cortisol can increase abdominal fat, so it will lessen glucose usage, raise your blood sugar, predispose you to diabetes, and its effects on calcium can increase osteoporosis.

So, be careful not to overdo it. Take breaks and listen to your body. Consider doing intense sessions later in the day, when cortisol levels are typically lower. Eat right to fuel your body immediately after exercise, to dampen the cortisol response. There are *herbal adaptogens* that can actually help improve your body's response to stress, such as tulsi or holy basil.

You don't need to spend an hour or more a day exercising to get results. Many experts have proven routines that help you reach your goals with thirty minutes of exercise. Pick the time of day that feels best for you, look at your calendar, and schedule the allotted time of your day that keeps other activities or daily chores from getting in your way. It is better to mix up your routine so it won't become boring.

You can start with something as simple as a walk, but make sure you add a weight-lifting routine eventually. It is necessary

10 Journal of Strength and Conditioning Research. 2002.

for fat burning, balance, and strength to lift weights at least three days per week. On those days you lift weights, spend ten minutes on interval runs or walks. This will help your strength building and cardio in a thirty-minute workout.

> *I am extremely pleased with the services that I have received from Total Approach Wellness. The medical and office staff truly care about helping their patients. I received expert advice and a custom treatment plan based upon my individual needs as well as exceptional support throughout my wellness journey. If you are serious and want to achieve great results and are willing to follow the expert advice, then I highly recommend Total Approach Wellness.*
>
> ~ Quentin C.

Conclusion

We intend this book to be a roadmap for you as you research health information, which is exploding at a monumental pace. Although the specifics may be outdated tomorrow, principles will not be. A lot of us are searching for the answers to our symptoms, such as fatigue, depression, unhealthy weight, hot flashes, loss of muscle mass, and stamina. We are dedicated to finding a reason for your symptoms. It is not enough to identify what is wrong; we will help you find out why this is happening.

Become empowered to take charge of your health. You have but one life, one body. Cherish it and nourish it. By protecting your health and taking a proactive approach, you can avoid many commonly occurring diseases.

In order to find out the *why,* you need to partner with a dedicated professional who looks out for your interest and will focus on finding you the relief you desperately need. Many of us suffer the same symptoms that modern medicine—with all its prescriptions and dedicated healthcare dollars from insurance and pharmaceutical companies—has failed to resolve for you. We want to find the answers with you.

No one person has all the answers; this is why we take a team approach to your journey to wellness. It takes a team of dedicated professionals to dig deeply into each individual's healthcare needs. We are dedicated to applying 100 percent of our knowledge, experience, and education, as well as our team of mentors, educators, and other committed, respected professionals toward identifying and resolving your healthcare needs.

Next Steps

We give you this book as a part of our Lifestyle Program. We challenge you to pass this along to someone you love and want to live a better, healthier, and more productive and abundant life.

We encourage you to call us at Total Approach Wellness and Aesthetics, 910-322-7368, email us at staff@tawellness.net, or visit our website TAWellness.net to learn more about us, Functional Medicine, and what we can offer you.

Please like us on Facebook at Total Approach Wellness and Aesthetics.

About The Authors

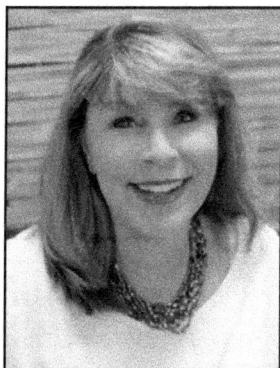

Cynthia Phillips is a board-certified physician assistant, co-owner of Total Approach Wellness and Aesthetics with Dr. Gerianne Geszler, and a fellow of Metabolic Medicine.

Cynthia's passion is to help people on their journeys to wellness. She has worked in an insurance-based practice for twenty-two years, and for the last ten years of that practice, she has been on the path to wellness medicine. She feels there are many people who need guidance to bring forth their wellness and change the sickness inside them. She wants to help people live a healthier, more vibrant life well into their nineties, or even hundreds, with an active mind and vibrant body to go with it.

She is dedicated to her patients' health and her own, mentoring them along the way. She has guided multitudes of people to successful weight loss as a beginning to their healthy lifestyle with the knowledge they carry to sustain this new lifestyle for the rest of their lives. She has guided many women through menopause and perimenopause and has guided many men to a more vibrant lifestyle with the help of testosterone replacement therapy.

Cynthia attended Wake Forest Bowman Gray School of Medicine, Campbell University and was awarded her bachelor of science. She also attended the Fellowship in Anti-Aging, Regenerative and Functional Medicine (FAARFM), American Board of Anti-Aging Health Practitioners, and is a Health Practitioner Diplomate. She gained the National Commission on Certification of Physician Assistants.

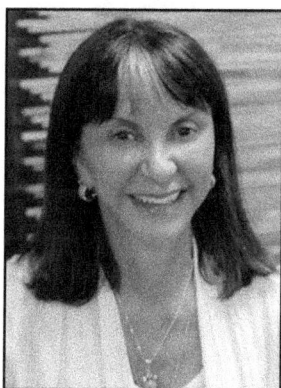

Dr. Gerianne Geszler is a gynecologist and a functional medicine physician. She actively practiced obstetrics and gynecology for twenty years after medical school and residency at Duke University. Her first love is hormonal balance, but she also has a passion for vibrancy and longevity, beginning with conception. Having provided maternity care for many women, she realizes the importance of a healthy vessel for a healthy baby to prevent problems in infancy and childhood.

This philosophy of care extends to the discipline of functional medicine, which focuses on addressing the root cause of illnesses that plague many as they age. She believes in a comprehensive, systems approach to the health problems she encounters. Dr. Geszler has presented workshops over the past ten years, and she has assisted many patients—both those struggling with healthcare issues and those who wish to age well.

www.ingramcontent.com/pod-product-compliance
Lightning Source LLC
Chambersburg PA
CBHW052053270326
41931CB00012B/2736